I0450620

Sleep Deep
Every Night

from the
Naturally Simple Health Series

by

Stephanie Yeh

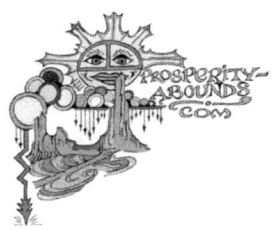

Contact Information: syeh@stephanieyeh.com
Visit my website: www.prosperity-abounds.com

<u>Disclaimer and Legal Notice:</u>

Sleep Deep Every Night

Sleep Hygiene Habits | Effective Tweaks

From the Naturally Simple Health Series

by Stephanie Yeh

Table of Contents

Sleep Deep Every Night

√ Sleep Hygiene Habits
√ Effective Tweaks

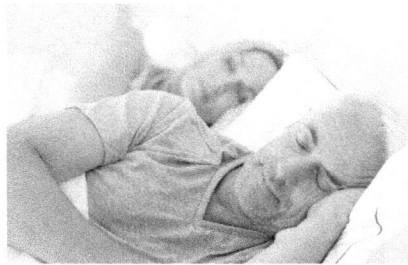

Avoid Watching the Clock. If you can't sleep, constantly checking the time or watching the clock will often increase your anxiety. Instead, get up and distract yourself. Drink some warm milk or decaf tea, read a book, or do some light house chores until you feel sleepy.
(health.com)

Get Rid of Worry Before Bed. Worry and stress can greatly increase your chances of sleeplessness. Dump your worry and stress before bed. For some, dumping worries into a written journal each night before bed can work wonders. Studies show that exercising for at least 10 minutes three to four hours before bed helps the body generate neurotransmitters and hormones useful for sleep.
(National Sleep Foundation)

Eliminate Stimulants. Stimulants in your food and beverages can prevent you from sleeping well at night. Because different people have varying reactions to stimulants, you will have to determine how stimulants affect your sleep. If you are sensitive to stimulants, avoid the intake of certain foods and beverages after noon. Beware of hidden caffeine, which can be found in chocolate, medications, weight loss pills, soda, and even some pain relievers.
(WebMD)

Can't Sleep?

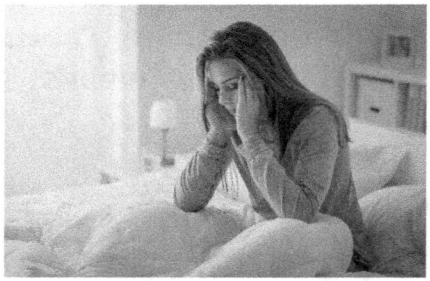

Join the Club!

Did You Know That ...

- **Stress is the top reason for insomnia, and more than half of all Americans lose sleep because of stress and/or anxiety.** (Mayo Clinic)

- **People sleep about 20% less than they did 100 years ago.** (Psychology Today)

- **A headache is no longer the top reason to avoid sex. Couples offer lack of sleep as the top reason for not having sex.** (Consumer Reports)

- **Statistics show that 100,000 vehicle accidents occur annually due to drowsy drivers. About 1,500 people die each year in these accidents.** (Nat'l Hwy Traffic Safety Admin)

- **About 10 million Americans consistently use prescription sleep aids, all of which have known side effects.** (National Sleep Foundation)

- **50-70 million adults in the U.S. have a sleep disorder, with 4.7% reported falling asleep or nodding off while driving at least once in the prior month.** (Sleep Association)

Sleep Deep: The Details

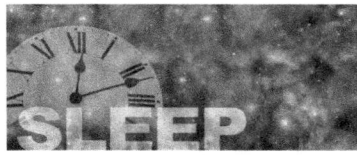

Are you tired of being tired all the time because you are unable to sleep as deeply as you wish? No worries. Understanding the mechanics of deep sleep can help you catch up in your ZZZs. Check out these uncommon tips for deeper sleep.

Uncommon Tip #1: Clock In and Clock Out
To keep your body on a regular schedule, use your clock wisely. Set an alarm to alert you that it is time for bed (or that it is time to prepare for bed by engaging in a soothing nightly ritual). Also set your alarm for the morning, and be sure to get up when your alarm rings in the morning. Be sure to set your evening and morning alarms for the same time each day. The more avid you are about following a regular schedule, the more likely you are to experience good sleep. Avoid hitting the snooze button, as snoozing can actually make you feel more tired rather than more rested when you get up.

Uncommon Tip #2: Soothe Your Inner Child
Bifidus, or Bifidobacterium bifidum, is a type of beneficial bacteria found naturally in the intestines. Some Bifidus supplements have added ingredients, such as bluegreen algae and the prebiotic inulin to nourish the Bifidus (check out Bifidus at gohealth.tips/bifidus). Bifidus is an important part of early childhood development, and strongly affects self-esteem, confidence, and sense of wholeness. Taking two to four Bifidus capsules before bedtime can help with waking up rested and confident.

Uncommon Tip #3: Pay Attention to Your Circadian Rhythm
Your circadian rhythm is your body's internal clock, which tells you when to sleep, wake up, and eat. This rhythm can be affected by factors such as sunlight, temperature, and hormones. In addition to using an alarm clock to help you maintain a steady

sleep cycle, you can help your body maintain a healthy circadian rhythm (thus getting enough restful sleep) by getting between 5 to 30 minutes of sun exposure without sun glasses as soon as you get up in the morning. This action tells your brain to wake up, and also affects the production of melatonin, a hormone that helps regulates the sleep cycle.

Uncommon Tip #4: Avoid Staying Up Late

Many who have difficulty with sleep mistakenly believe that staying up late will lead to better sleep later in the night. Studies show that staying up late simply keeps the brain engaged so that you will fight a brain buzz as you try to fall asleep later. Instead, follow a regular sleep cycle rather than trying to "tire yourself out" to get a good night's sleep.

Uncommon Tip #5: Make and Keep Meaningful Connections

Staying connected with people who are meaningful in your life can stave off conditions of aging such as disrupted sleep cycles or Alzheimer's. In fact, studies show that loneliness can negatively impact sleep patterns, blood pressure, immunity, and emotional health. Staying social, on the other hand, "appears to enhance health, and may even increase longevity," says Thomas Perls, M.D. Some preliminary studies indicate that online social media can have similar social impacts.

Uncommon Tip #6: Shut Down Blue Lights

Most of the electronics that we use every day emit blue light, which is a frequency of light that can disrupt or prevent sleep. To avoid sleep disruption from blue light, power down electronics such as TVs, smart phones, digital clocks, and e-readers for several hours before bed. You can also wear orange-tinted glasses to block out blue light, use apps available for your smartphone, computer, and tablet to prevent screens from emitting blue light. Finally, block out all sources of blue light in your bedroom such as digital clocks or a smartphone left charging overnight.

Get Your Free Consult for Sleeping Deep & Learn More about Healthy Lifestyles

Visit gohealth.tips/consult to get your free Deep Sleep Consult from Prosperity-Abounds.

Common Sense Tips for Deep Sleep

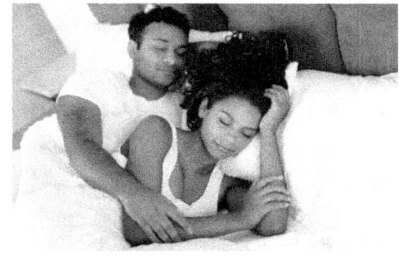

Looking for more ways to increase your beauty sleep? Check out the following common-sense suggestions for better sleep.

Common Sense Tip #1: Limit Naps

Napping is a logical way to get a quick boost of energy when you are tired. But limit the number of and length of your naps, since napping too long or too frequently can often interfere with your ability to fall asleep at night. Many studies show that naps lasting no longer than 20 minutes are the most effective for boosting energy and mood while not interfering with your ability to sleep at night. Also, avoid napping too late in the day.

Common Sense Tip #2: Limit Activities in Bed

Limiting your activities in bed to sleep and sex can really help you sleep better at night. This practice is called sleep hygiene. Sleep hygiene is the removal of habits and outer stimulus that interferes with a person's ability to fall asleep or stay asleep during the night. These might include watching TV right before bed, eating or drinking right before bed, exercising before bed, and more. People who practice good sleep hygiene are much less likely to suffer from poor sleep. Read more about sleep hygiene in the Resources section.

Common Sense Tip #3: Check Your Posture in Bed

If you suffer from back or neck pain, you may be suffering from poor posture in bed. If you have lower back pain, sleeping on your side and placing a pillow between your knees can ease your back. Sleeping on a firmer mattress can also improve your posture in bed, plus ease low back pain. For neck pain, check whether your pillow is causing your head and neck to be out of alignment. Try different pillows until you find one that keeps your head and neck in a neutral and aligned position. Your neck is in a neutral position if your nose is aligned with the center of your body.

Common Sense Tip #4: Check with Your Doctor
Because certain medical conditions and medications can affect your sleep patterns, ask your healthcare provider whether any aspect of your health could be contributing to your lack of sleep. You can help your healthcare provider diagnose you by keeping a sleep diary for a week or two. Note nights when you cannot sleep, the number of hours you sleep each night, the number of times you awaken each night, and whether you wake up refreshed in the morning.

Common Sense Tip #5: Use a Soothing Bedtime Ritual
Studies show that creating and strictly following a bedtime ritual can often cause poor sleep patterns to diminish or even disappear. Following a regular bedtime ritual helps regulate your body chemistry so that you more easily fall asleep at around the same time each night, and also wake up refreshed around the same time each morning. These rituals can include taking a warm bath, using biofeedback, listening to soothing music, drinking warm milk, or exchanging foot rubs with your significant other.

Common Sense Tip #6: Skip the Snooze Button
As tempting as it might feel to hit the snooze button in the morning to catch an extra three to five minutes of sleep, studies show that the little sliver of sleep you get during the snooze cycle actually makes you feel more tired, not less. According to Robert

Rosenberg, D.O., this kind of "fragmented sleep can result in moodiness, cognitive problems, and trouble paying attention." To retrain your body to stop snoozing, Rosenberg suggests strategies such as putting your alarm clock out of reach so that you have to get out of bed to turn off your alarm.

Bonus Tips for Deep Sleep

Need Some Quick Tips?

Desperate for sleep? Check out these overlooked tips that can help you sleep more deeply.

- **Allergy-proof Your Bedding and Mattress**: If you consistently sneeze, sniff, cough, or snore when you are in bed, you may be allergic to allergens in your bedding and mattress, including dust mites, mildew, dander, and more. Limit your exposure to these allergens, cover your pillows, mattress, and box spring in zippered covers that separate you from these allergens. The best covers are made of microfiber. Change and wash bedding at least once a week in hot water. If you have pets, keep pets out of your bedroom to prevent the accumulation of dander.

- **Avoid Heartburn**: Many people are kept awake at night by heartburn. This is often the result of eating too large a meal too late in the day. In addition, poor digestion can contribute to heartburn. Avoid this problem by eating a smaller dinner at least three to four hours before you plan to go to bed. Take digestive enzymes with your meal to aid in digestion. Finally, sleep on your left side, a posture that studies indicate reduces heartburn.

- **Make Your Sleep Environment Comfortable:** Consider the factors that promote easy sleep for you. Studies show that sleeping with socks helps some people. Other people cannot sleep when the temperature is too high. Listening to soothing music or white noise in the background helps some people fall asleep and stay asleep. Experimenting with different pillows can help you find the best pillow for your body.

- **Soothe Your Senses:** Aromatherapy has been shown to provide inner tranquility and, for some, faster sleep. The most popular essential oils to promote sleep include lavender, bergamot orange, ylang-yang, lemon, sage, and clary. Add a few drops to your bath, use an aromatherapy diffuser, or add essential oil to a carrier oil and rub it directly onto your skin.

Rediscovering Sleep

"I have not slept well or deeply for many years. It turns out I had a few bad habits that kept me from sleeping soundly each night. The changes that helped the most included taking Bifidus before bed, kicking Fred (my cat) out of bed so I could stretch out, and unplugging from blue-light electronics an hour or so before bed. I would not say that I sleep deeply every night, but I do sleep much more easily and much more deeply than I have since I was a child."

~ Joe Davidson, San Diego, CA

Deep Sleep Success Profile

Profile: Betty Dunne, age 29

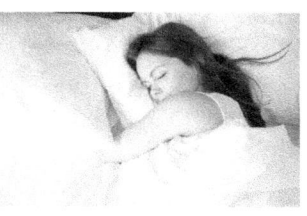

Goal: Get deep quality sleep at night despite a history of poor sleep patterns.

Strategy for Success: After consulting with her doctor, Betty decided to use several strategies for better sleep.

- **Clock In and Out**: Betty used a clock to help her go to bed and get up in the morning at the same time each day. This consistency helped her body follow a more regular schedule for sleeping and waking.
- **Adopt a Sleep Routine:** Since Betty prefers taking baths to showering, she took a scented bath each night before bed. She also listened to soothing music and went to bed wearing socks (proven to help some people sleep better).
- **Move Sherman the Dog:** Because Betty's pet dog, Sherman, consistently took up a lot of bed space, Betty bought him his own bed so she could stretch out in her bed.
- **Exercise in the Evening**: Taking a brisk walk every evening at least three to four hours before bed helped Betty unwind from her day so she felt more relaxed at bedtime.
- **Improve Posture in Bed:** After trying several pillows, Betty found that a pillow filled with barley was the most comfortable for her head and neck.
- **Unplug:** After learning that the blue lights from electronic equipment can interfere with sleep, Betty turned off all electronics at least an hour before bed.

Results: By using a variety of strategies, Betty found that she slept better than she had in years. While she averaged only five to six hours of sleep per night, she was able to sleep more soundly each night. She also felt more alert in the morning, even without the help of coffee, and had more stamina during the day. Betty continues to experiment with her sleep environment for even better results!

Frequently Asked Questions About Sleeping Deep

Is it true that lack of sleep can be life threatening?
YES. Studies show that lack of sleep can contribute to car accidents, poor job performance, relationship issues, mood disorders, memory loss, heart disease, obesity, diabetes and more.

What is insomnia?
Insomnia is the habitual inability to fall asleep or stay asleep. According to the National Sleep Foundation, there are multiple types of insomnia:

- **Acute**: A brief period of sleeplessness often caused by a stressful life event
- **Chronic:** A consistent pattern of being unable to fall or stay asleep three or more days per week
- **Onset:** The inability to fall asleep at the beginning of the night
- **Maintenance:** The inability to stay asleep, waking up often and then being unable to fall asleep again.
- **Co-morbid:** Insomnia that occurs with other conditions, such as anxiety or depression.

What are the symptoms of insomnia?
People who suffer from insomnia can experience symptoms that include difficulty falling asleep (often for hours at a time), unrestful sleep, frequent periods of wakefulness, and waking up too early. Insomnia is the most common sleep disorder in the U.S., and up to 95% of people in the U.S. report at least one episode of insomnia. Insomnia becomes a problem when a person experiences these symptoms chronically or for a limited period of time when experiencing high levels of stress.

What is a normal sleep cycle?

To attain restful sleep, a person needs to experience a normal sleep cycle. A person's normal sleep cycle has two categories: REM and non-REM. REM is rapid eye movement. During REM sleep, a person experiences muscle relaxation, periodic rapid eye movements, and dreaming. Non-REM sleep has four stages, which range from light sleep to deep sleep. A normal sleep cycle has about 75% of non-REM sleep, and 25% of REM sleep. People who suffer from insomnia have disrupted sleep cycles, which leads to a lack of restful sleep.

How many hours of sleep does a person need?

Sleep requirements vary from person to person. On average, studies show that adults need an average of seven to eight hours of sleep each night to feel rested. Teenagers may need up to nine hours of sleep per night, and infants need a whopping 16 hours of sleep every 24 hours.

What can I do if I cannot sleep?

- Get out of bed
- Don't stress about the time or number of hours of sleep you get
- Use any of the tips in this book to restore your sense of calm
- Exercise patience... erasing bad habits can take time. Give your body time to adjust to a new and healthier sleep regimen (one month for every year you have had poor sleep hygiene)

Can I make up for lost sleep?

No. Just get back to your regular sleep cycle as soon as possible.

Resources for Sleeping Deep

One of the best ways to get to sleep, stay asleep, and wake rested is to practice what is called "good sleep hygiene." Sleep hygiene is the practice of removing anything (habits or outer stimuli) that prevents a person from falling and staying asleep, or feeling rested from sleep. Some recommended tips for sleep hygiene include:

- Use the bed only for sleep and sex. Do not participate in other activities while in bed, including watching TV, working, or eating.

- Avoid eating or drinking right before bed. Also avoid the following in the hours just before going to sleep: spicy foods, a large meal, excessive alcohol, (alcohol may help a person fall asleep, but often results in the person waking up just a few hours later), and caffeinated drinks (coffee, tea, or soda).

- Exercise can help you sleep, but exercise at least three to four hours before bed.

- Eat healthy snacks if you are hungry at night. Do not eat anything for at least an hour before bed. Snacks that are easy to digest and helpful to eat before bed include cereal and milk, or cheese and crackers.

- Avoid participating in activities that cause you to think for at least an hour before bed. These activities may include watching TV, using your phone or computer, playing video games, or working. Instead consider reading a book, meditating, listening to soothing music, or taking a warm bath.

- Get adequate exposure to sunlight during the day, and also ensure that your sleep environment is dark at night. Light and dark cues help your body produce the appropriate hormones for sleeping and waking.

- Make your sleep environment comfortable. Check on factors such as light, sound, temperature, sleep clothing, sleep rituals before bed, and more. For instance, many sleep studies have shown that sleeping in a quiet environment is helpful, but having too much quiet can actually amplify sounds such as a dripping faucet or a barking dog in the distance. Some people sleep better if they wear socks to bed. Vary the temperature at night until you find a temperature range that is most conducive to deep sleep for your body and personal preferences.

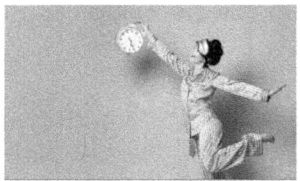

Deep Sleep Hacks from Real People

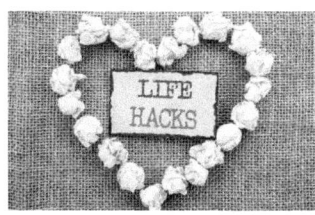

Follow My Nose

"I have played around with and studied aromatherapy for years. One of the reasons that aromatherapy is so effective is because, of all the senses, the sense of smell has the most direct path to the brain. To tempt myself out of bed I set either my coffee maker or my aromatherapy diffuser to start ten minutes before I want to get up. That way, when my alarm goes off, I wake up to the great smell of coffee, peppermint, or cinnamon, all of which make me feel happy! When my nose is happy, then I am happy to get out of bed (or at least happier than without the tempting smells!). This also means I am more comfortable going to sleep and resting deeply. I know I will have a solid sleep followed by a delightful wake up scent!"
~ Ethel B., Crystal Falls, AK

Play Goldilocks

"I never had trouble sleeping until a couple of years ago. I could not find any reason for my poor quality of sleep. I didn't want to use sleeping pills so I tried all kinds of alternative methods. Nothing really worked. One of my friends suggested I get a new mattress or try an air mattress with variable firmness. First, I tried a new regular mattress (after testing a dozen or so at the mattress store). At first the mattress seemed to result in deeper sleep, but after a few weeks I was restless again at night. Next, I added a memory foam layer to my mattress. Again, I slept better for a while, but then failed to sleep well again. Finally, I decided to splurge on an air mattress with adjustable firmness. Guess what? Goldilocks (that's me) is finally happy. It turns out that I need different levels of firmness in my mattress depending on whether my body is sore from working out or tired from sitting in front of a computer all day. Even if I wake up in the middle of the night, I can tweak the firmness of the mattress and go right back

to sleep. My sleep hack? Get a mattress that can be adjusted to suit your moods and body condition. It's worth every penny!"
~ Curtis R., Magnolia, DE

Feed the Body and Brain
"When I was having trouble sleeping, I went to my go-to guy, my acupuncturist. Without going into his long explanation, his short version was that I didn't have enough fuel in my body to sleep. I thought this was weird because usually when a car runs out of fuel, it stops. I figured that when my body ran out of fuel, I would either be hungry or tired. Not so. Apparently, the body and brain both need certain kinds of nutrients and energies to repair and rejuvenate at night. When these are lacking, the body and brain sometimes can't shut down. In addition to acupuncture treatments, my Doctor of Chinese Medicine suggested I take some supplements to fuel my brain and body so I could rest at night. For my brain he suggested some micro-blended bluegreen algae (see gohealth.tips/AFAMicro) that had the right mix of nutrients to support brain health. For my body he suggested the whole algae cell (see gohealth.tips/AFA) with plenty of glycogen and other nutrients for physical support. It took about three months for me to start sleeping well. The good news is that I have not had any trouble sleeping since I started this regimen, no matter what is happening in my life."
~ Scott Y., Kouts, IN

White Chestnut and Mimulus Flower Essences
"I am a chronic worrier. Even when I was a kid, I would replay the day's events over and over in my head before I finally fell asleep out of sheer exhaustion. I struggled with this problem well into adulthood, when my repetitive thoughts were compounded by worries and fears. I found no relief until a friend suggested I try some flower essences or other vibrational remedies. Since flower essences are fairly harmless if they don't fit the problem, I chose this alternative method to try to calm my mind at night. The internet was truly helpful in helping me figure out which flower essences would work best. After playing around I settled on White Chestnut (for repetitive thoughts) and Mimulus (for known

fears). I have taken them every night and they have helped me with many nights of peaceful rest."
~ Mindy L., Groveland, GA

Act Like My Cat
"No excuses but I have not treated my body the best when I was younger. That means when I wake up in the morning, I am always stiff and often pretty sore. Plus, I often wake up in the middle of the night when various aches and pains in my body announce themselves. Not good. So, I decided to follow my cat's example. She is the most flexible being I know, and she never wakes up stiff and sore. She stretches all parts of her body before settling in for sleep, and prior to getting up. I do what I call "bed yoga" before I go to bed. It's no formal kind of yoga, but I stretch out different parts of my body by feel, until I feel loose and warm. Then I roll over and go to sleep. The results are amazing. I still wake up feeling my age, but my body is way less sore and achy than it used to be. I also tend to sleep through the night most nights. I call my approach 'Cat Bed Yoga'!"
~ Taylor W., Plano, TX

Bifidus to Sleep Like a Baby
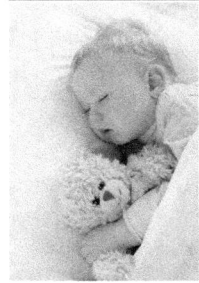
"When I got promoted into a new high-stress position at work, I was thrilled. I also stopped sleeping well at night because I felt insecure. Luckily my friend is a doula, and she suggested I try taking this probiotic called Bifidus (beneficial bacteria that lives in the large intestine—see gohealth.tips/bifidus). It's the probiotic that protects infants from birth through about two years of age. Apparently, babies who lack this probiotic often feel insecure, while babies who have plenty of this bacteria are reported to be more content. I started taking a few capsules of a guaranteed-live strain of Bifidus at night before bed, and after a week I started sleeping better. After a month I found I slept better than I had in a long time. It makes sense to me... if it works for babies, why not for me?"
~ Vicki D., Huntington, NY

Take a Bath for Rest, and a Shower to Wake Up

"Generally speaking, I'm a shower person, especially in the morning when I want to wake up and get going. I used to take a shower at night, too. But one Christmas I made bath salts (Epsom Salt and Lavender essential oils) as gifts. I made some for myself as well, so I decided to start using them regularly. The first few nights I took a warm bath at night with my Lavender Bath Salts, I was pretty amazed at how well I slept. I thought maybe I was just tired from long hours at work. But even when I caught up on sleep, taking a bath with aromatherapy continued to bring me good sleep. I decided to read up on it, and discovered that the warm bath relaxes the body, and then the drop in body temperature after the bath matches the body's natural process as it prepares for sleep. So now I get it. I don't take a warm bath every night, but it is definitely my go-to solution whenever I want to definitely have a good night's sleep!"
~ Daris M., Jersey City, NJ

Meditation, My Way

"For better sleep, I have tried more traditional forms of meditation in the past—even joined some meditation groups, but I confess that I was never really able to calm the chattering monkey in my mind to settle down. Then I learned about something called "tracing." Basically, when I lay down in bed to sleep, I calm my mind by starting with feeling sensation in my right hand. Then I move that sensation up my arm, across my shoulders, and down my left arm. Then I keep moving the sensation in a continuous path around my body until I fall asleep. Theoretically, I should be able to send that 'feeling of sensation' all around my body but I find that I fall asleep long before I get very far. Sometimes I start with the sensation in my foot or even in my big toe. All the different ways I could play with this form of meditation makes it fun... makes it meditation MY way. Best of all, I fall asleep quickly and tend to stay asleep most nights."
~ Amy E., Santa Ana, CA

Stop Playing Tug-of-War

"I love my husband dearly but I have to say that he is a total blanket hog. No matter how equally the blankets are shared at

the beginning of the night, within a couple of hours I find I am shivering under a thin sheet while my hubby is buried under a mound of blankets. So, guess what? I decided to stop pulling the blankets back over... several times each night. Instead, I got my own blanket that covers just me. We sleep in a king size bed and I used blankets made for a double bed. I lay them over my side of the bed only, and I have never had to play tug-of-war again! I now sleep soundly through the night under my very own set of blankets!"
~ Leslie F., Greensboro, NC

The "Stop Snoring Sleep Shirt"
"My wife has complained about my snoring since the day we got married. She has tried earplugs, kicking me awake, and all manner of other methods to get me to stop snoring. One day she presented me with her version of the "Stop Snoring Sleep Shirt," which was a T-shirt with a tennis ball held in a pocket sewed into the back of the shirt. She said that I always snored when I lay on my back, so the tennis ball should solve that problem... and it did! Granted, I had a few bruises on my back for the first week or so, but after that I got into the habit of sleeping on my side. The funny thing is that not only did my wife sleep better, but I slept better as well."
~ Drew S., Mesa AZ

Old-Fashioned Books
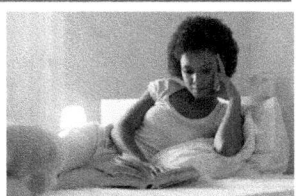
"I've always found reading soothing but I find that if I read a book on my computer tablet at night, I get progressively more awake, not sleepier. So, I've returned to old-fashioned books. Maybe it's my age but I find something soothing about holding a real book in my hands and turning pages. I've also heard that electronics put out a kind of light that keeps our brains alert. Whatever the reason, there is nothing that guarantees me a good night's rest than a good paperback from one of my favorite authors. I buy these books by

the dozen at my local thrift store, and call it the cheap and easy solution to excellent rest!"
~ Ginger H., Chesapeake, VA

Sleep Despite Creaky Aching Joints
"At age 72, I remain a committed weekend warrior. I love working out with my weekend cycling group, I play pickle ball most weekends, and I work hard to keep my yard in shape. In the summer time, I also water ski and swim on a regular basis. My joints are my weakest link, and I sometimes have trouble sleeping if my joints ache after a particularly strenuous weekend. Luckily, I take a joint supplement (see gohealth.tips/joints) that helps protect and support my joint cartilage, and a mix of proteolytic enzymes (see gohealth.tips/enzymes2) to reduce the effects of over-exertion. Whenever I think I might have overdone it, I take both supplements. I have found that this preventative measure helps me sleep well at night... and helps me stay the weekend warrior that I love being!"
~ Will K., Verona, KY

A Laundry List of Things to Avoid
"I'm a major DIY gal when it comes to quality of life. I went through a phase where I researched the quality and length of my sleep, using a sleep tracker bracelet and phone app, because I discovered the multiple health benefits of deep, restful, and satisfying sleep. In my efforts to get that quality of sleep, I added and subtracted all manner of items from my life. I researched what others had tried, experimented on myself, and recorded my results. I have boiled it down to a laundry list of things to avoid to sleep better at night. For my best night's sleep, I avoid:
- heavy exercise at least three hours before bed
- more than one glass of wine at dinner
- heavy meals for dinner (I eat my heaviest meal at lunch)
- drinking too many liquids after 6 p.m.
- viewing any electronic screens (including the television) at least an hour before bed

- caffeine of any kind after 3 p.m.
- staying up past 10 p.m. (the body starts rejuvenating at around 11 p.m. according Traditional Chinese Medicine)"

~ Nancy R., Oklahoma City, OK

Chill Out and Put on Socks!

"Some of my friends think I'm weird, but I sleep better if I keep my bedroom cooler than many people, around 62 to 64 degrees Fahrenheit... and go to sleep with socks on. I used to have a roommate who slept with the temperature up around 70 degrees Fahrenheit and I could *not* sleep at all. Once she moved out, I put the thermostat back down to my comfort zone, and put on my socks! Anytime I sleep in a hotel, I try to adjust the temp to my comfort zone, and I never forget to pack my socks. There is something about general cooling but toasty toes that keeps me at maximum happy slumber. If I had to advise someone else, I would say that the trick is to find the right combination of temperature and clothing that promotes your best sleep."

~ Tasha S., Walla Walla, WA

Get Your Free
Deep Sleep Consult

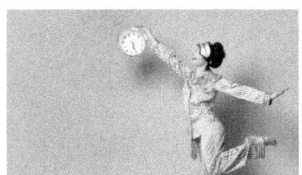

About the Author

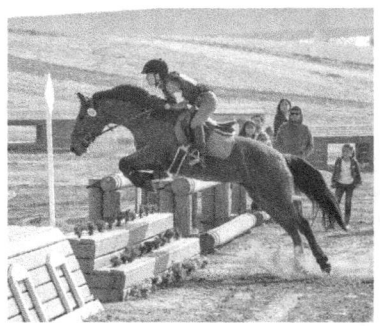

Stephanie Yeh has been researching, learning, and publishing about natural health solutions for over 20 years. Her interests include the use of whole foods, natural supplements, herbs, flower essences, homeopathics, vibrational healing, Edgar Cayce remedies, and bodywork for people and animals.

She has partnered with a wide variety of people to create vibrant natural health for people and their pets.

Stephanie is super passionate about horses and their health, and has enjoyed helping many rescued equines regain health and happiness.

Stephanie enjoys sharing her knowledge of natural healing through a variety of channels, including:

Website: www.Prosperity-Abounds.com

Blog: Prosperity-Abounds.Blogspot.com

Nutritional Consultations: gohealth.tips/consult

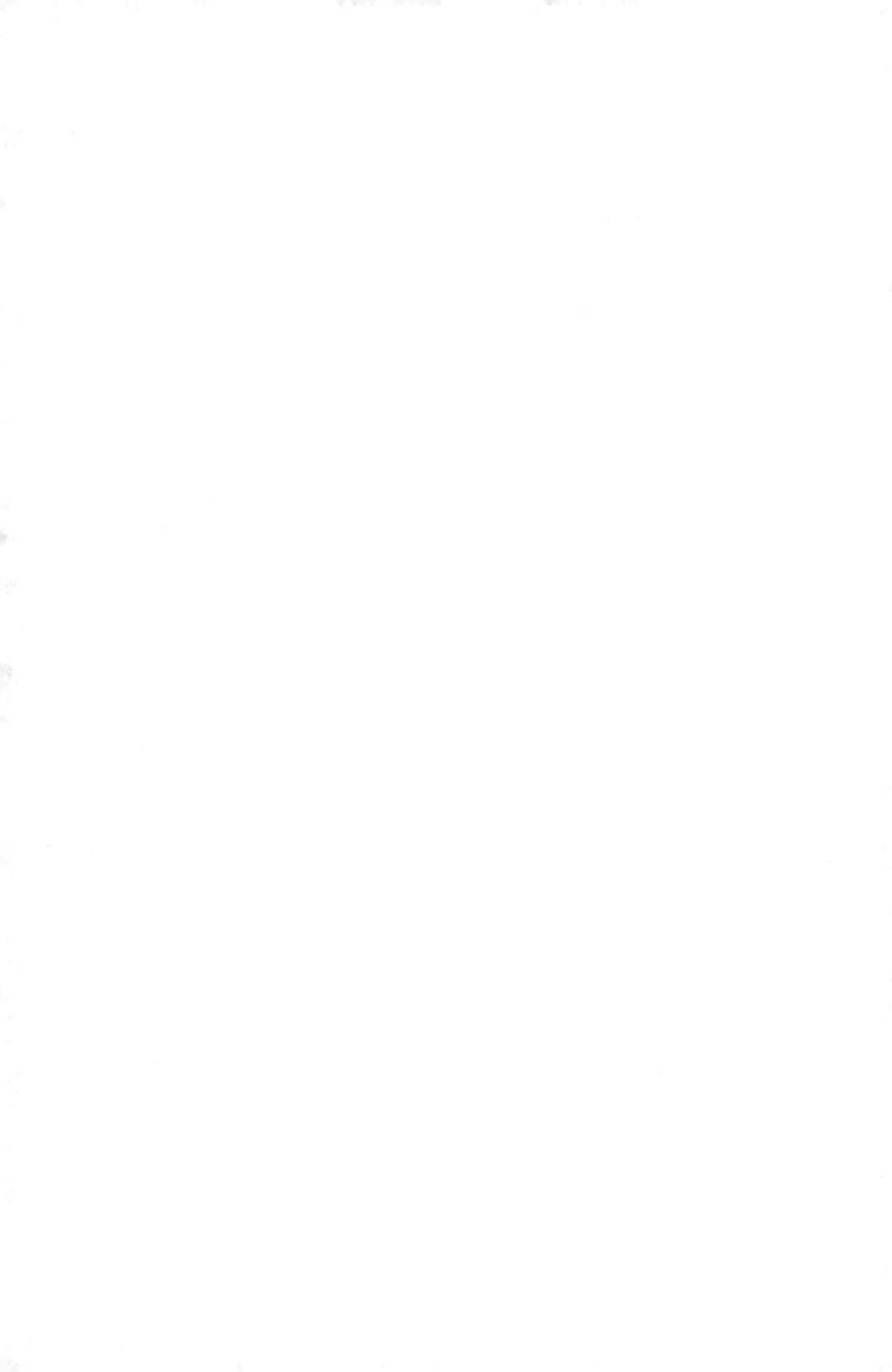